D0358195

A GOOD HEALTH GUIDE

The Diabetic's Guide to Healthy Living

Maxwell Stein

The Diabetic's Guide To Healthy Living
Maxwell Stein

This edition published MMIII by The Windsor Group
The Old School House,
1 St John's Court,
Moulsham Street,
Chelmsford,
Essex CM2 0JD

© Copyright MMIII The Windsor Group

Typeset by SJ Design and Publishing, Bromley, Kent

ISBN 1-903904-02-1

Contents

Introduction

Throughout literature from the earliest times, there are references to a mysterious disease, which was accompanied by the passing of large amounts of urine and other life threatening symptoms. Early Greek physicians called this disease 'diabetes', which meant 'flowing out' or 'fountain'. Combine 'diabetes' with the Latin word 'mellitus', which means 'honey' or 'sugar', and 'diabetes mellitus' becomes 'fountain of sugar'.

Much research was carried out by the 17th century English physician, Thomas Willis, who made the discovery that the urine of sufferers of this disease was sweet. This was done by the obvious process of tasting the urine, which he discovered was 'wonderfully sweet', as if it contained honey or sugar!

It was another hundred years, however, before another English physician, Dr. Dobson, carried out various experiments with the urine of such sufferers and noticed that their urine fermented like alcohol; he, therefore, came to the conclusion that the sweetness observed by Willis was due to sugar, a fact which he was later able to prove. This sugar, which we know to be dextrose and glucose, comes from the carbohydrate or starchy materials which we consume as food, with a certain amount coming from the protein parts of the diet as well.

We now know what this mysterious disease is, and have found many ways to fight it. But to understand diabetes, we must first consider the normal process of food metabolism. Several things happen when food is digested. Sugar called glucose is extracted from our food and is released into the bloodstream for distribution to our muscle and fat tissues where it can be used as fuel. To aid the transfer of glucose from the blood stream, the pancreas manufactures insulin, which has the role of promoting the transport of glucose across the plasma membranes of cells.

In insulin deficiency, muscle cells are deprived of glucose and begin to utilise alternative energy sources. Thus, fat and protein reserves of the muscle tissue are utilised for oxidation and energy production, resulting in wasting of muscles, weakness, and weight loss. Weight loss is further worsened by what happens in the fat cells of the adipose tissue. Not only can glucose not enter these cells, but the loss of insulin removes the inhibition of the enzyme 'hormone-sensitive lipase', resulting in increased breakdown of stored triglycerides and mobilisation of fatty acids.

To understand the effects of diabetes, the author has applied much energy in researching the disease to find ways in which to combat the problems that it creates. As a result, this book is his contribution to help sufferers to understand the importance of diet and exercise as an aid to good health and well-being.

Its purpose is a practical one. It has been planned and

written with the all important view of showing how a simple and concise programme of diet and exercise can improve your lifestyle. Everything you do to help yourself to stay healthy will help you on the road to leading the sort of life you want to live. It will also help you to avoid the health problems associated with diabetes in later life.

It is hoped that this book will prove to be of great practical value and interest, and will also serve as a helpful guide to the best ways of maintaining good health, and understanding the discipline of diet and exercise. By applying the programme to your daily activities, you can automatically raise your quality of life and in so doing enhance every day you live.

Chapter One

Diet and Blood Sugar Control

Good diabetes control means keeping your blood sugar level as close to normal as possible. The difficulty of keeping to a sensible diet is that we tend to think of dieting regimes as insipid, and that fad foods, or comfort foods as they are so often called, are tasty. Many people who like to have more than a few pints at their local each day often say, "What the hell, we only live once." Well, how wrong can you be! You may only live once, but it will be a short life, and a very disagreeable life at that.

Let's face it, if you don't follow a reasonable diet then you will be heading for all sorts of trouble. As if obesity isn't enough to put up with, there are all sorts of other problems in store. And that message is not only for diabetes sufferers but anyone who ignores the danger signals. Still not impressed? Well let me tell you! If you suffer from diabetes, then in the short term high blood sugar, (hyperglycaemia) or extremely low blood sugar (hypoglycaemia) can lead to dizziness, mental confusion, unconsciousness, and even death. Then there are other complications like heart disease, kidney failure or nerve damage. Some sufferers go blind or develop gangrene, which means the loss of a limb. I could go on, but I think that's enough of that, so what about the good news?

Fortunately diabetes doesn't have to be as dire as the disease is painted. There are rational methods and means at your disposal to help you lead a healthier, more active life. First of all though, you have to accept the fact that there is no standard or special diabetic diet, that we are all individuals, and we all have our own dietary requirements. Having said that, there is a lot of wholesome dietary advice given in these pages that you can follow to help control blood glucose and lipid levels. After all, it is a far healthier way of life for us all to consider.

KEEPING BLOOD GLUCOSE LEVELS UNDER CONTROL

Regular testing is the only way of knowing whether or not your blood glucose levels are in their target range. When away from home, carry alcohol swabs or moist tissues to wipe your fingers prior to testing when necessary. Keep a daily record of injections, medications and test results. If you have trouble with your blood glucose levels, follow the adjustment guidelines as discussed with your doctor or diabetologist for advice. Be sure to have your documented list of medications handy to help the doctor provide appropriate care.

SELF TESTING

There are testing devices you can use yourself, such as the 'Accu-Chek Advantage' available over the counter at most pharmacies. It is specifically designed for easy use, and to reduce the pain of testing through a combination of a test strip, finger pricker and a meter. The advantage of using such a device is simple. You can use it in any location, at any time. Only a tiny drop of blood is required, and when the test strip is inserted into the meter, it automatically gives a blood glucose reading in seconds. At the same time, ensure that your blood pressure and cholesterol are checked regularly.

TRIAL OFFERS HOPE FOR INSULIN PILL

Researchers in Israel are claiming an early success in the quest for an insulin pill, which could one day replace the need for daily injections for over half a million UK citizens who suffer with diabetes. The work, which is in its very early stages has yet to be tested on people with diabetes. In the first stage of testing the pill will be tried out on patients with Type 2 diabetes, and if successful trials will be extended to include patients with Type 1 diabetes.

Mairi Benson, Information Science Manager at Diabetes UK is reported to have said, "The difficulty with insulin is that it is broken down in the stomach before it can get into the bloodstream to do its job. This is why it currently has to be injected rather than taken in tablet form. This early success in overcoming this problem is encouraging but there is still a long way to go before we know if it will be safe and successful."

Myth

My friend says that type 2 diabetes is a mild form of diabetes, so I needn't do anything about it!

Your friend is totally wrong. There is no such thing as mild or borderline diabetes. Any form of diabetes is serious, and if not properly controlled can lead to serious complications.

Chapter Two

Developing A Healthy Diet

By eating the right foods and maintaining a healthy weight people who already have diabetes can take an active role in controlling the condition and preventing serious complications. With the right diet, many people with type 2 diabetes can reduce or eliminate their need for insulin. You and your dietician should work together to design a meal plan that is right for you and make sure that it includes foods that you enjoy. A diabetes meal plan is a guide that tells you how much and what kinds of food you can choose to eat at meals and snack times.

One of the problems with diabetes is that it makes you want to eat more. To solve that problem, and the ensuing problems overeating brings, space your meals throughout the day. Instead of having large meals once or twice a day, try eating a small breakfast and then a small snack a couple of hours later. Then take a small lunch and a small dinner with a snack in between at similar intervals. Timing of meals and snacks is important, so as to maintain a relatively consistent carbohydrate-protein-fat intake pattern from one day to another. At the same time, meal plans allow for a variety of menus, to allow for a wider selection of foods to be consumed without straying too far from the recommendations of the plan.

A meal plan doesn't dictate which specific foods to eat for a meal, but it does tell approximately what time to take the meal, which food groups to refer to when planning the meal's menu, and identifies the number of servings to take from each food group.

Making-up meal plans is invaluable in maintaining good blood sugar control, because it is a strategy to help keep dietary carbohydrate (protein and fat, too) consistent, so that the best medication-activity-diet balance can be identified and better achieved. A good meal plan should fit in with your schedule and eating habits. The right meal plan will also help keep your weight where it should be. Whether you need to gain weight, lose weight, or stay as you are, your meal plan can help.

CARBOHYDRATES

Not so long ago we were told by nutritionists that foods such as bread, pasta, potatoes, and rice were fattening, stodgy and generally not good for us. Nowadays, we are told that we should be eating more of them, as they are an essential part of a healthy diet. The simple truth is, the experts got it wrong. When you look at the consumption of carbohydrates on a global scale they amount to about 75% of people's total calorie intake. However, in the developed world they comprise only 45% of the diet. Ideally, carbohydrates should provide 50% of your daily diet, mainly in the form of pasta, brown rice, potatoes, and wholemeal bread.

The useful role of carbohydrates is now widely recognised, and many experts believe that if foods containing carbohydrates are consumed throughout the day as evenly as possible, there will not be the vast swings in blood sugar levels as previously encountered when eating fatty, sugary foods. This is particularly important to people with diabetes. Many people with diabetes who take short-acting insulin can learn to adjust their insulin to match their carbohydrate intake. We call this an insulin-to-carbohydrate ratio.

A measure of how quickly the energy from a carbohydrate is made available for use as energy is the glycaemic index.

Food Type	% Glucose Conversion	Time Taken
Simple Carbohydrates	100 %	15 to 35 minutes
Complex Carbohydrates	90 - 100 %	30 to 95 minutes
Protein	60 %	3 to 4 hours
Fat	10 - 30 %	More than 4 hours

COUNTING CARBOHYDRATES

Dieticians, diabetic associations, and freelance writers have all devised or written about new methods to help you count carbohydrates. Optimistically, I hope each and every one has been of help in providing a successful tool. However, there is a very simple method for counting carbohydrates, and that is done by reading the list of ingredients on the labels of the products that you buy. Since it became compulsory for food manufacturers to list the contents on food labels, you will see under the heading

'Nutritional Information', a line that shows the total number of 'Carbohydrates' per serving. With this method, you can keep a check on the carbohydrates you are going to consume, and act accordingly with your medication.

FOODS CONTAINING CARBOHYDRATES

- breads
- cereals
- cookies/cakes/pies
- grains
- honey/syrup/molasses
- ice cream/frozen deserts
- pasta
- rice
- potatoes
- crackers
- sucrose (table sugar)
- fruit/fruit juice
- soda pop/sweet beverages
- jam/jelly/preserves
- vegetables
- milk/yogurt

LOOKING AT HEALTHY FOODS

We all know that no single food will supply all the nutrients our body needs, so good nutrition means eating a variety of foods. If we divide food into four main groups we will be better able to understand why it is important to eat something of each group each day.

Fruits and Vegetables

Plant food provides plenty of fibre and may therefore help lower blood sugar and blood fat levels. Most fruits and vegetables can be bought fresh all the year round. Exotic produce arrives from Africa, South America, Israel, and Europe; they all arrive on the supermarket shelf, as fresh as the day they were picked. Many of the larger stores display leaflets on their shelves. These will often explain all the information needed with reference to description, taste and nutrition, and also give details of how to cook and store safely.

Eating plenty of fresh or frozen fruits and vegetables will give you the fibre and vitamins that your body needs. If the produce has been grown organically, leave the edible skins on, this will add extra fibre to your diet. But, do make sure that the skin is washed before eating. Aim for at least five portions a day to provide you with sufficient vitamins and fibre as well as to help you balance your overall diet. A portion is, for example, a piece of fruit or a serving of a vegetable.

Vegetables are better consumed when they are steamed or raw, as generally they raise blood glucose levels more slowly than when they are peeled, cooked, mashed, marinated, or had sauces added to them.

Potatoes can be cooked in a variety of ways, and are included in one out of every three meals eaten in Britain today. When prepared in a wholesome way, potatoes are a great source of energy and pack a nutritional punch.

Apart from sweet potatoes and sweetcorn potatoes are the only starchy food to supply a substantial amount of vitamin C, and a useful amount of vitamin B_1. In fact, one medium potato has 45% of the vitamin C recommended daily for good health. Potatoes are high in fibre and carbohydrates and contain more potassium than a banana. They are naturally low in calories and contain no fat, sodium or cholesterol.

People think of potatoes as fattening, but that is wrong, the real culprit is the fat that they are often cooked in, or which is added at the table in the form of butter or cream. Potatoes are best cooked by boiling, steaming, baking or microwaving. Add only small amounts of 'unsaturated margarine, low fat sour cream or yoghurt products to keep your meal healthy.

When refrigerating or freezing potatoes – it turns the potatoes' starches to sugar and will cause potatoes to turn dark when cooked. Store potatoes in a cool, dark and well ventilated place. Too much light will cause them to turn green, and make them inedible.

Dairy Products

Most people tend to overeat on dairy products, which is a sure way to increase body fats and cholesterol, so be moderate when eating these products. By dairy products I mean, cheese, milk, and eggs, and the by-products made from this produce. Limit the number of eggs you eat to three or four a week. When eating eggs, make sure that they are cooked right through so that the yolk as well as the white are solid. Avoid commercial foods containing raw eggs, these include ice cream, eggnog, mayonnaise, many brands of salad dressing and Hollandaise sauce. Some dressings use pasteurised eggs which are OK. Choose monounsaturated fats, e.g. olive oil and rapeseed oil. Use diet margarine making sure that it doesn't contain hydrogenated vegetable oil. Drink skimmed milk rather than full fat. Choose low fat dairy foods like low fat yogurt.

When storing fresh dairy products refrigerate at 5° C. or below and remove from the refrigerator just prior to cooking. When purchasing, look for products that are not past their 'sell by' dates which are marked on the packaging and use the before the 'use by' date.

Meat And Fish

Protein is needed for growth and provides energy for you muscles to work on. Healthy choices include lean meat products. That is meat with the extra fat removed, also, when eating poultry, make sure the skin is removed. It's important to try and cut down on the fat you eat, particularly saturated (animal) fats, as this type of fat is linked to heart disease. Eating less fat and fatty foods will also help you to lose weight. Grill, steam or oven bake instead of frying or cooking with oil or other fats.

Fish provide so many important nutrients that they should form a major part of your diet. Not only is fish tasty, but it's also an important source of vitamin B_2, fluoride, iodine, omega-3 oils, and iron. In fact, fish is packed with protein without excessive calories. Even the fattiest fish contain far less fat and cholesterol than most cuts of red meat.

As important as it is to know how to select a safe variety of fish, it's also vital to make sure that your choice is fresh. When selecting fresh salt water fish it should have a mild ocean smell, whereas, fresh, fresh-water fish smells like cucumbers. fresh fish will have bright eyes, and a bright red colour under the gills. The skin will glisten and when pressed shouldn't leave an indentation.

Avoid all fish that are dull or limp, have red, sunken eyes, and a strong fishy or ammonia odour. Also, avoid any fish that shows frost damage; it may indicate that it's been stored for a long time or has been thawed and then re-frozen.

When buying ready cooked shellfish the shells should be intact and the shellfish should feel heavy for their size. Poor quality shellfish may contain liquid if the shells are cracked before cooking. So check by shaking them gently. If not already shut, live shellfish should close when tapped. Cooked prawns and shrimps should always be firm and pink in colour.

Male crabs have larger claws than females, so there is more white meat in them. On the other hand, female crabs have more and better quality dark meat inside the shell. Crabs should move when touched. Lobster should curl their tails under when picked up.

Grains

Carbohydrates give you energy. Eat regular meals based on starchy foods such as bread, pasta, potatoes, rice bran, and cereals. This will help you to control your blood glucose levels. Whenever possible, choose high fibre varieties of these foods, like wholemeal bread and wholemeal cereals, as fibre maintains the health of your digestive system, and prevents problems such as constipation. It's best to spread the consumption of grains out during the day.

Brown unpolished rice is healthy grain that contains 'b-sitosterol', a naturally occurring substance which lowers blood cholesterol, and can help insulin-dependent diabetics to normalise their blood sugar levels.

Beans and Lentils

Dried beans and lentils, or pulses are a popular, tasty, healthy food. The list of produce is extensive, it includes black-eyed peas, chickpeas, lentils, and black, red, white, and kidney beans. Not only are they versatile, they are well worth eating, especially in place of higher fat meat or cheese. Pulses provide many of the nutrients the human body needs, such as protein and carbohydrates. In addition, the iron, folic acid, calcium, magnesium, potassium and B vitamins found in pulses help meet daily vitamin and mineral requirements.

Pulses which are rich in soluble fibre, can substantially reduce blood cholesterol rates, which helps reduce the risk of heart disease. Many studies confirm that eating pulses, can improve blood sugar control. Pulses slow down the rate of digestion and result in a more gradual rise and fall in blood sugar, steadying energy levels.

Comparing Pulses (¹/₂ cup cooked legumes)					
	Calories (g)	**Protein (g)**	**Fat (mg)**	**Iron (mg)**	**Calcium**
soybeans	86	14	8	4	88
lentils	100	9	1	3	19
kidney beans	88	8	1	3	25
black beans	41	8	1	2	25
Chickpeas	82	7	1	3	40

(Source: American Dietetic Association)

To replace the protein in a meal, use 55 grams dry weight of pulses per person. To reduce cholesterol and blood fat levels, 100 grams of pulses, dry weight, a day is ample.

Tip

It is said that drinking sage tea in conjunction with insulin treatments may help boost insulin action. However, before adding it to your diabetes management plan, discuss it with your doctor.

LOOKING AT NOT SO HEALTHY FOODS

Fat

Fat may be an unhealthy choice, but because it is a nutrient, you do need some fat in your diet. However, too much fat won't do you any good at all, and it can be very harmful to people with diabetes.

One of the major problems with eating too much fat is that it may increase the chances of heart disease and/or hardening of the arteries. Unfortunately, people with diabetes have a greater risk of developing these diseases than those without diabetes. So it is very important that you limit the amount of fat in your diet.

WHICH FOODS ARE HIGH IN WHICH FATS				
Saturated fats	Skin on poultry Fatty meat	Butter Cheese	Sausages Pies and pastries	Lard Dripping
Monounsaturated fats	Olive oil	Olive oil Spreads	Rapeseed oil	Peanuts and peanut oil

Polyunsaturated fats	Salmon, trout, herrings, mackerel	Polyunsaturated spreads	Sunflower oil	Corn oil
Omega-3 oil	Mackerel, herring, salmon	Walnuts and walnut oil	Rapeseed oil	Soya products and soya bean oil
Omega-6 oil	Brazil nuts, walnuts, sunflower seeds	Sesame oil and peanut oil	Sunflower oil	Soya products including tofu

- Instead of butter on bread, trying using polyunsaturated spread.
- Instead of cooking with corn oil, try using rapeseed or virgin olive oil.
- Instead of making salad dressings with sunflower oil, try walnut or peanut oil for a change.
- Instead of eating fatty meats, try eating fish containing plenty of omega-3 oil.
- Instead of eating rich desserts, try eating lots of fruit instead.

Salt

Using lots of salt in your food can raise your blood pressure. Many commercial foods contain too much salt. Sometimes, you can taste it – as in pickles, bacon, quiches, and ready cooked meals. There is also a lot of hidden salt in other foods, such as cheeses, salad dressings, and canned soups. Remember, when using salt – a little goes a long way. Try flavouring food with herbs and spices instead of salt.

Sugar

People with diabetes should eat less sugar. So cut down on sugar and sugary foods. This does not mean you need to eat a sugar-free diet. Sugar can be used as an ingredient in foods and in baking as part of a healthy diet. However, use sugar-free, low sugar or diet squashes and fizzy drinks, as sugary drinks cause blood glucose levels to rise quickly. Foods high in sugar include: desserts, icing on cakes, sugar frosting on patisseries, sugary breakfast foods, table sugar, honey, and syrup. One 200 millilitre can of regular soft drink contains two teaspoons of sugar.

Drinks With Hidden Sugar

Most sweetened soft drinks provide plenty of energy, but no other useful nutrients. These are known as 'empty calories'.

Every year in the UK, we consume about 8.25 billion litres of soft drinks, comprising fruit juice, waters and carbonated drinks.

Per 200ml	Sugar in grams	Calories
Coca-Cola	21	86
Diet Coca-Cola	Nil	0.9
Diet orange drink	1	3

Per 200ml	Sugar in grams	Calories
Lemonade	11	42
Lime juice cordial	10	58
Lucozade	37	152
Orange squash	10	36
Ribena	24	98
Rosehip syrup	21	77
Tonic water	11	50

Myth

I am told that should I refrain from eating sweets and chocolate; is this true?

There is no reason why you shouldn't eat sweets provided they are eaten as part of a healthy diet, or combined with exercise. Also, if you are taking tablets or insulin to treat your diabetes, you may at times need to eat high-sugar foods to prevent your blood glucose levels falling too low.

Myth

People say that you will get diabetes if you eat too much sugar. Is this true?

The answer is a definite NO! Diabetes is caused by the failure of the pancreas to manufacture sufficient levels of the hormone insulin. However, if you have a history of diabetes in your family, or you are overweight, the risk of developing Type 2 diabetes is increased. The risks are also increased if you have a history of Gestational diabetes (diabetes in pregnancy), are over the age of 40, or you are of Afro-Caribbean or Asian origin.

Alcohol

The best advice is: stay away from alcohol. But, if you like an alcoholic drink now and then, drink in moderation only – that's two units of alcohol per day for a woman and three units per day for a man. For example, a small glass of wine or half a pint of normal-strength beer is one unit. Here are some guidelines to keep in mind if your choose to drink:

☐ Never drink on an empty stomach, as alcohol can make hypoglycaemia (low blood glucose levels) more likely to occur. Blood glucose levels are at their lowest levels overnight, and drinking without eating may cause you to experience delayed low blood glucose during the night.

☐ Only drink when you have someone with you who can assist in case of an emergency.

☐ Alcohol and alcoholic mixers contain calories and must be counted as part of your daily allowance.

☐ Use low-calorie diet mixers or low-calorie sodas with your drinks.

☐ Avoid fortified beverages such as liqueurs, and fortified wines, which all have a high sugar content.

☐ When drinking socially, alternate alcoholic drinks with diet soda or water, and sip drinks slowly to avoid a rapid rise in your blood glucose level.

Caffeine

Caffeine, like alcohol, is a drug. It doesn't contain calories, and has no nutrient value at all. Many people regard drinking coffee which contains caffeine as an important part of their daily ritual. They claim that it keeps them awake and on the ball. Admittedly, in moderation, it can increase alertness and boost your energy level. But, caffeine does affect the central nervous system and in excessive amounts, can have a very negative effect on stress management. The ability to recover (calm down) after a stressful event is greatly impaired with caffeine. The more caffeine, the more pronounced the effect.

Stress management is an important health skill to acquire. Hormones of stress (glucagon, adrenaline) raise blood sugar. The longer one is under stress, the longer these counter-regulatory hormones are active. This effect can make blood sugar more difficult to control.

Individual tolerances to caffeine vary. Most people are advised to consume no more than 500 mg of caffeine daily. This would be the equivalent of 4 small cups (not mugs) of coffee. Less is best.

When cutting down on caffeine, be aware that you may experience withdrawal symptoms such as headaches and fatigue. Cutting back gradually over 2 to 4 weeks can help to minimise this problem.

Chapter Three

Eating Sensibly

In general, you should follow the same guidelines for eating sensibly as everyone else. If you do this, you will find that planning your menus and selecting foods in the right amount at all difficult. Once foods have been organised into lists, balancing selections between carbohydrate, protein and fats, and measuring food portions is easy.

To begin with, limit your fat consumption to less than thirty per cent of your calories each day. Say no to saturated fats, (these are fats that are solid at room temperature) and eat more polyunsaturated fats. Ways to reduce fat consumption include choosing lean cuts of meat and trimming extra fat. Eat more fish and poultry (without the skin), and drinking low-fat or skimmed milk.

Plan your diet to include twenty per cent of the calories from protein sources, such as dairy products, meats, poultry, vegetables, and fish. Remember that some of these foods can be high in fat, so choose carefully with the advice of your doctor or dietician. If you have kidney disease, you may need to limit protein to ten per cent of calories.

Get up to fifty per cent of total daily calories from complex carbohydrates. Foods such as beans, vegetables, and grains (such as breads, cereals, noodles, and rice) have a strong affect on blood sugar. Eating the same amount of these foods from day to day can help keep blood sugar at a steady level.

Plan meals at consistent times, so that blood sugar is more stable. This also helps insulin work better.

Use alcohol with caution and never on an empty stomach. Alcohol can cause very low blood sugar.

Myth

I have been told that I should restrict the amount of starchy foods in my diet. Is this correct?

No. Until the 1970s, diabetics were advised to follow a high-fat, low carbohydrate diet. However, since then, increasing evidence has shown that carbohydrates, such as bread, potatoes, cereals, rice and pasta are helpful in reducing coronary risk, and help to keep blood glucose levels steady. Wholemeal or wholegrain starchy foods are also a good source of fibre, which helps keep your gut healthy.

CASE STUDY

For Maureen, getting the children off to school on Monday was a hurried affair, causing her to skip breakfast. When Maureen arrived at work she wasn't her usual cheery self, and became quite aggressive and uncooperative when greeted by her co-workers. By ten o'clock Maureen was staggering around as though drunk and behaving irrationally. Her supervisor knew that she was an insulin-dependent diabetic and called the company nurse, who recognised that her symptoms might indicate hypoglycaemia. Maureen was taken to the company surgery and was persuaded to drink a glass of sweetened milk and eat a slice of bread, thus providing slow-acting carbohydrates to stop her blood sugar level from falling even lower. Within half an hour Maureen had returned to her normal self. Maureen told the nurse that she had a cold coming on, and hadn't had time to eat any breakfast, although she had taken her usual morning dose of insulin. The nurse explained that her uncontrolled, drunken symptoms was caused by her blood sugar level plunging because she had taken the insulin and not following it with some food.

EATING OUT

Eating in hotels and restaurants could be a sure way to break your willpower to follow a well executed plan for healthy eating. Fortunately, a typical diabetes meal plan consists of foods that are generally available in most restaurants.

Virtually any food offered in restaurants can be incorporated into your meal plan, provided you exercise some restraint on excesses. Managing your food consumption away from home involves estimating appropriate amounts of the foods offered. Try to keep your calorie intake close to your typical level unless you are more active than usual. With the help of your dietician, you can vary the types of food you eat. For example, you can try different sources of carbohydrate. Monitoring these changes can help you keep your meal plan on track and may help ward off potential problems.

Always have some snacks with you in case your blood glucose level drops or you're unable to eat your next scheduled meal on time. Cheese and crackers, fresh or dried fruit, and sandwiches are all healthy choices that are easy to take along in a carry-bag, picnic basket or cooler. Also take some quick-acting sugar with you, such as glucose tablets or juice.

FOOD SAFETY

Food poisoning can be especially dangerous to people with diabetes. In the United Kingdom about two million people a year suffer from an attack of diarrhoea and/or vomiting due to food poisoning. Most do not consult their doctor and the cause is not often found. Many raw and perishable foods contain toxin-producing bacteria or parasites. When these foods are undercooked or are handled, prepared or refrigerated improperly, dangerous levels of these organisms can develop. One of the most common bacteria found (about 40,000 cases annually) are called Campylobacter found in raw poultry and in unpasteurised milk. Salmonella multiplies rapidly at room temperature – or outdoor temperatures in the summer. It affects about 30,000 cases annually. They may be present in raw meat, poultry, and occasionally eggs. For the remainder, Staphylococcus Aureus, Clostridium Perfringens, and Bacillus Cereus produce toxins or poisons in food which may result in severe vomiting.

Some types of food poisoning can produce symptoms with a few hours of the contaminated food being eaten, whilst others may not occur for some. People who have food poisoning may think they have the flu, because the symptoms are similar: diarrhoea, vomiting, fever, chills, headache and muscle cramps. In most cases, symptoms are fairly mild and subside within a day. Some cases of food poisoning, though, grow more severe or include blood in the stools, if so, see a doctor right away.

PREVENTION IS BETTER THAN CURE

No one is saying that you mustn't eat those foods commonly implicated in food poisoning, since Salmonella, Campylobactor and E. Coli 0157 are destroyed in foods during cooking, provided they are adequately cooked. But, before you unpack your shopping, or pack your coolbox for a day out, here are a few tips to ensure that your foodstuff is remains wholesome and untainted:

- ☐ Prevent the growth of bacteria by ensuring that your refrigerator is covered and adequately chilled to around 5° C.
- ☐ When shopping, don't leave chilled or frozen foods too long in the boot of your car. If a long journey is involved keep the produce in a coolbox that is well iced, and don't pack it too full.
- ☐ Wash hands, surfaces and utensils before and after handling uncooked meat. Particularly when handling other foods.
- ☐ Take care to ensure thorough cooking and re-heating of all meat, especially poultry.
- ☐ Make sure that deep frozen food is thawed before cooking. This is especially important when using a microwave oven.

☐ Keep uncooked meats in sealed containers so juices don't spill on other foods in the refrigerator or when transporting them.

☐ Buy vinegar-based salads if mayonnaise-based varieties can't be kept cold.

☐ Thoroughly wash all produce with cool water before cooking and eating.

☐ Store marinated meats in the refrigerator.

☐ Boil marinades for ten minutes before pouring over cooked foods.

☐ Avoid eating raw eggs or uncooked foods to which they have been added.

☐ Do not drink any kind of unpasteurised milk.

Your Diet In Practice

It's so easy to make excuses for not keeping up your eating plan. You can blame your friends for a start, because it isn't always easy to maintain a diet, especially when you are pressured into going for binge or rave-up with them. But unless you are prepared to stick to your diet, you won't make any progress at all. Ask yourself, in all honesty, is good health worth giving up for the sake of going on a binge?

Unfortunately we can't have our cake and eat it. The idea that we can have an occasional binge and stay healthy is a non-starter. Future illness can only be avoided if your diet becomes an ongoing regime. If you really want to keep healthy, then you must be prepared to change your outlook, and diet for life.

VITAMIN D AND DIABETES

Could a lack of vitamin D be the cause of type 2 diabetes in postmenopausal women. A new study in Italy has shown a possible link between type 2 diabetes, which generally strikes older people, and reduced levels of vitamin D. Researchers report that other experiments have linked reduced vitamin D-binding proteins with insulin deficiency. A study of nearly 800 postmenopausal women was carried out to determine the occurrence of vitamin D deficiency and dietary calcium insufficiency. Each patient underwent a test to determine their vitamin D level, and were then asked to complete a questionnaire about their calcium intake. During the tests, each patient was asked, in detail, about their daily activities. The reports were then assessed for inclusion in the report.

The results of the tests found that women with type 2 diabetes had considerably lower levels of vitamin D and had a much lower dietary calcium intake. Researchers say that they have no data to explain the prevalence of vitamin D deficiency. But, it is thought that the reason for the reduced intake of calcium could be because overweight diabetics are urged to reduce their consumption of diary products.

Researchers are still working on their findings, and suggest further studies are needed to establish the importance of vitamin D deficiency in the progression of type 2 diabetes.

GINSENG AND DIABETES

The September issue of *Diabetes Care* reports that in a randomised, placebo-controlled study, researchers gave capsules of North American ginseng (Panax quinquefolius) to diabetic subjects who were already receiving treatment for diabetes in the form of diet or prescription drugs.

To obtain a result, researchers gave some of the patients a 3g dose of ginseng and others a placebo at varying times of up to 2 hours prior to taking a blood test. The results were wholly rewarding. Blood tests revealed that the patients who had been given ginseng had a blood sugar level that was 59.1% less than patients who had received the placebo treatment, regardless of the time the dose was given. disappointingly, further tests with doses above 3g did not improve on the results already achieved.

Research by other facilities indicates that ginseng may assist in treating forms of dementia by helping to restore short term memory, and enhance concentration and cognitive abilities, which may be impaired by improper blood supply to the brain. The adaptogenic qualities of ginseng helps to balance the body, depending on the individual's needs. It is reported to normalise blood pressure, increase blood circulation and aid in the prevention of heart disease. Ginseng has been used as an aid in the treatment for diabetes, radiation and chemotherapy protection, colds, chest problems, to aid in sleep, and to stimulate the appetite.

A word of caution before you decide to buy a supply of ginseng. Ginseng should be only be used therapeutically with the consent of your doctor or hospital diabetologist. Although subjects in the study did not report major side effects, ginseng can potentially augment the effect of prescription drugs used to lower blood sugar, causing a dangerous decrease in blood sugar. There may also be adverse effects if taken at the same as oral anti-diabetic drugs, such as Warfarin, heparin, aspirin, and NSAIDS.

Chapter Four

Diabetes and Your Health

All types of diabetes are serious diseases, and each type can lead to the same complications. However, there are many things you can do to stay healthy. Eating a healthy diet, and increasing your physical activity is a good start, but there are other things you can do that are just as important, such as learning as much as possible about diabetes and its consequences. To do this you must involve your doctor, hospital diabetologist, and dietician. These are the professionals who can tell you what to do, and arrange for you to have regular tests to check for the complications of diabetes. Remember, these tests are important to you and your future health, so make sure you are getting the best possible care.

DIABETES AND MALE IMPOTENCE

If you are a man, you may find it hard to get a good erection. Unfortunately, this is a very common difficulty in men with diabetes. If this is your problem, you should definitely see a doctor, preferably a specialist that your doctor will refer you to for assessment. Don't be shy about talking to your doctor about it; you never know, there may be something that will help you to solve the problem. Usually the most common cause of impotence is just anxiety – and not necessarily because you are diabetic.

Don't ever think that impotence is the end of your world; there are many ways to overcome this problem using various medications and mechanical aids. One of the most successful drugs to overcome impotence in recent years is Viagra (sildenafil). This is effective in up to 60% of diabetic patients. Before taking the drug it is important to discuss its possible side effects with your doctor. Side effects include: flushing of the face, headache, indigestion, blocked nose, dizziness and a short-term bluish tint to the man's vision. Viagra does not automatically cause an erection, this will only happen when the man is sexually stimulated. It also takes time to work, so it needs to be taken about one hour before intercourse. A word of warning to users of this drug – it is very powerful, and should never be taken casually.

Scientists are constantly researching new drugs to combat impotence and Uprima is one worth mentioning. Uprima was placed on the market on 21st June 2001, at a considerably lower price than Viagra. It is administered by placing it under the tongue and letting it dissolve; in this way, it works much faster than Viagra.

Mechanical aids have been around for a long time. The 'Pubic ring' and the 'Vacuum pump' are both claimed to be effective for men who can't maintain an erection for very long. Unfortunately with the latter, the penis tends to look blue in colour, and feels cold to the touch.

There are many helpful benefits available from the world of herbal healing. Ginkgo is supposed to increase the blood flow into the penis, as also does Cardamom. It is best taken by adding two bruised cardamom pods to a cup of coffee. The Californian herbalist Kathi Keville, author of *The Illustrated Herb Encyclopædia* and *Herbs For Health And Healing*, recommends steeping ten grams each of Oats (Avena Sativa), ginkgo leaves and ginseng root in half a litre of boiling water. Let the brew cool and strain before drinking.

Whatever form of treatment you may decide is best for you, sex counselling is a must. Because impotence may be entirely due to psychological causes, it is essential that you put off any course of treatment until you are certain what the problem is. It may be that counselling alone can bring about a cure. But even if the problem is physical, counselling is often necessary as a supplement to the main treatment.

The National Health Service provides a limited budget for drug therapy which means that only certain patients can receive treatment on the NHS; fortunately diabetics are among those listed.

If you need further help, contact one of the following:

The Impotence Association. Helpline: 0208 767 7791.

Family Planning Association. Helpline: 0845 310 1334.

Brook Advisory Centres. Helpline: 08000 185023. This service is only for young people who are 25 and under.

WellCare Lifestyle Clinics. Freephone 0808 100 3133

DIABETIC RETINOPATHY

Diabetic retinopathy is an eye disease usually resulting from either diabetes mellitus or alternatively from persistent hypertension. There are three classes of retinopathy:

background retinopathy, maculopathy and proliferative retinopathy. These are not different diseases but are a spectrum of the same condition which means that a person may change from one type to another over time.

If left untreated, diabetic retinopathy can lead to blindness, and can occur in connection with all types of diabetes, regardless of whether it is treated with tablets, insulin, or by diet alone.

What Causes Diabetic Retinopathy?

Diabetics have a higher chance of developing diabetic retinopathy, due to prolonged periods of high blood sugar levels, which causes haemorrhaging of the small blood vessels in the retina at the back of the eye.

Initially blood begins to leak from the blood vessels and may then congeal and obstruct the normal flow of blood. The bleeding then leaks into the retina, which may cause the retina to become swollen. To make matters worse, once the blood in the broken blood vessels congeal, the retina becomes starved of oxygen, which may then lead to the growth of new abnormal blood vessels on the retinal surface. These new abnormal blood vessels are fragile and bleed readily, consequently, haemorrhaging into the vitreous humour may then occur, enabling fibrous tissue to grown forwards into the vitreous humour.

Diagnosis

The diagnosis of retinopathy is made by an examination of the back of the eye by an ophthalmologist, or by your own doctor, if he/she is looking after your diabetes. During an eye examination, the ophthalmologist checks the external appearance, eye movement, visual acuity, visual field, and colour vision. The retina is then examined to assess its condition.

Have You Had Your Sight Checked?

Because the vision is not usually affected by diabetic retinopathy until it is at a very advanced stage, regular eye examinations need be carried out regularly to detect any disease before it can become beyond treatment. All people with diabetes should have their eyes examined at least once a year. If there is any evidence of retinopathy, your doctor will probably refer you to an Eye Clinic where the condition of your sight will be monitored at frequent intervals.

Prevention or Cure

The sooner you start controlling your blood sugar levels, the better the chances of preventing retinopathy ever happening. Prevention depends on the proper control of your diabetes. As this is not entirely a preventable disease, it is clear that long-term good diabetic control will help to reduce the amount of retinopathy.

Have Regular Check-ups – You need to be seen by an eye specialist who will dilate your pupils and check for signs of eye disease. Your regular doctor cannot do this special test in his or her surgery. Regular annual check-ups by a hospital diabetologist and ophthalmologist is very important to ongoing good health. In the long term, if diabetic retinopathy has already been diagnosed, as long as it has not reached an advanced stage, good control of blood glucose will prevent it from developing further.

STOP SMOKING

It is important not to smoke. In England alone, 111,000 people die per year from smoking related diseases. That's the equivalent of a jumbo-jet crashing every day, with no survivors! In fact, 40% of smokers die before retirement. In other words, 5.2 million needlessly die before the age of 65.

If you are a smoker then the overwhelming evidence of its detrimental health effects will be obvious to you. The following methods may help you to cut down, or stop altogether.

Acupuncture – will help, provided your really want to stop. Specially made needles are usually inserted painlessly into the addiction and lung points on your outer ear. Your practitioner may also insert small needles in your ear, which can be left in place, so that you can stimulate the points yourself, whenever you feel the need for a cigarette.

Naturopathy – is a natural way of overcoming addiction to nicotine, which incidentally, raises blood pressure, and speeds up the hardening of the arteries. Your practitioner will draw up a plan based on diet, relaxation and exercise specially suited to your circumstances. This will probably include dietary supplements, such as daily doses of vitamin C.

Hypnotherapy – is proving to be of very great value in therapeutic work. Hypnotic suggestion can also be used in conjunction with other forms of therapeutic treatment, and in many cases, enables a hypnotherapist to treat cases successfully when all other methods of treatment have failed. Hypnotherapy is pleasant and causes no side effects. The hypnotherapist gives suggestions to strengthen your resolve to stop, and reminds you of the harm smoking does to your health. Post hypnotic suggestions are implanted whilst you are still in a semi-conscious state, and will have a lasting effect.

BENEFITS OF VITAMINS AND MINERALS

Some evidence suggests that the following supplements may help prevent retinopathy: bilberry, vitamin C, and vitamin E. Vitamin B_6 and magnesium may also be helpful.

Vitamin B_6 – Researchers say they have seen a possible link between vitamin B_6 deficiency in patients with retinopathy. Observations gathered over periods ranging from 8 months to 28 years indicated that there was less incidence of retinopathy in patients with diabetes who happened to take vitamin B_6. However, there is still no direct evidence that vitamin B_6 can help.

Because vitamin B_6 is water soluble, you may take supplements containing more than the standard recommended dose; as the excess is lost from the body in urine. A typical safe therapeutic dosage of vitamin B_6 is in the range of 1.5 to 2 mg daily.

Vitamin C – Vitamin C plays a major role in the growth and repair of connective tissue, skin, ligaments, and muscles. Researchers have found that levels of vitamin C are lower in people with diabetes than in non-diabetics, and lower still in diabetics with retinopathy. This does not necessarily prove anything, but it does give grounds for more research. A deficiency of vitamin C may make blood vessels more likely to leak, and even if vitamin C isn't deficient in the whole body, it may be deficient in the eye, due to local conditions. The standard recommended dose of vitamin C is in the range of 10 mg daily. High doses of vitamin C should only be consumed with other antioxidants, such as vitamin E, because each vitamin keeps the other in a proper non-oxidised state.

Vitamin E – As an antioxidant, vitamin E helps to neutralise potentially damaging free radicals in the body, which may be useful in the fight against diabetic retinopathy. This fat-soluble vitamin has potent antioxidant effects on fat-soluble tissues like cell membranes; and it also has important blood-thinning effects.

It has been found that levels of vitamin E is lower in people with diabetes than in non-diabetics, and especially low in diabetics with retinopathy. This is a similar finding to that regarding vitamin C, and many of the functions of vitamin C with respect to retinopathy apply to vitamin E as well.

Some researchers have found that vitamin E raises already high blood pressure in some people. As a precaution, always monitor your blood pressure when you begin taking supplemental vitamin E, particularly since high blood pressure has been linked to retinopathy. Vitamin E also has the potential to thin the blood, so seek a physician's advice before combining it with other blood thinning medications.

The recommended daily allowance of vitamin E for an adult is in the range of 10 milligrams daily.

Bilberry extract – comes from a shrubby perennial plant from northern Europe and North America. This plant has a long history of use in the treatment of diabetes and its complications. The active substances in bilberry extract are known as anthocyanosides, which appear to have a special affinity for the eye, particularly the retina. These components appear to act as antioxidants in the body thus helping to strengthen connective tissues, such as that found in the retina, they also decrease the leakiness and fragility of the blood vessels.

Manganese – is stored in the liver, kidneys and pancreas. It is not strictly an 'essential' mineral, as the body can substitute other minerals for it if it is not present in the diet. But, because manganese is involved in the body's ability to cope with fats and glucose, manganese may help those with vulnerability to heart disease or to diabetes. There is no recommended daily allowance specified, but adequate supplies can be found in nuts, pulses and fruits. Wholemeal bread is another good source.

LASER TREATMENT

Since its invention in the 1960s the laser has become a very useful tool for treating patients in conditions where surgery can become unmanageable. The laser is a device which amplifies an input of light, producing an extremely narrow and intense monochromatic beam of light which can be applied to the back of the eye causing burns (or coagulation). It is applied in many tiny individual burns which destroy small areas of the retina.

Before applying laser treatment, some drops are put into the eye to make it feel numb, thus making the whole process quite painless. It may take between 50 to 2000 burns to complete the treatment, after which, the patient will be allowed to go home.

Side Effects

Laser treatment is usually carried on an 'out-patient' basis, after which, most patients will go home and observe no side effects at all. If, however, a lot of laser treatment is required then the peripheral, or side vision, may be affected. On rare occasions this may lead to a problem with night vision, or interfere with driving.

SURGERY

Although surgery is a drastic measure, it may have to be performed when the condition of the eye is very bad. This may be done if there has been copious bleeding into the eye from the abnormal blood vessels. It may also be necessary if laser treatment has been ineffective, or 'proliferative retinopathy' has been picked up at a late stage. This type of surgery is called 'vitrectomy.' It involves removing the jelly from the back of the eye and any bleeding is removed at the same time. Laser treatment may be applied at the time of the operation.

Myth

I am told that people with diabetes eventually go blind, is this true?

Agreed that diabetes is the leading cause of blindness in people of working age in the UK, but it doesn't mean that you will go blind. Research has proved that you can reduce your chances of developing diabetes complications – such as retinopathy – if you keep control of your blood pressure and glucose levels.

DIABETIC NEUROPATHY

Current estimates suggest that worldwide there could be thirty million people with diabetes. That's a lot of people, thus making it a safe bet that a lot of them have never heard of 'neuropathy'. The dictionary says that neuropathy is a common name for diseases of the peripheral nerves, usually causing weakness and numbness. And that's it in a nutshell, so now, you can forget about it. Not on your life! In the real world, regardless of whether the condition is acute or chronic, nerve disorders for diabetic patients are potentially serious ailments. In fact, diabetics who fail to take enough care in controlling their diabetes stand the highest risk of developing this disease; so be alert to the problems, and take notice of your doctor's advice.

Cause and Symptoms

Diabetic neuropathy is caused by a prolonged high blood glucose level. Once the blood glucose levels rise above a certain point, the nerves throughout the body gradually begin to be damaged. If you have symptoms such as burning, tingling, and numbness in your hands or feet, see your doctor and arrange for your hospital diabetologist to test you for neuropathy. Fortunately if the diagnosis is acute neuropathy, it will possibly disappear when your diabetes has been brought under control. But for those with chronic neuropathy there are more serious implications.

Neuropathy can affect the nervous system in several ways. It can lessen the control of your muscle functions making it difficult to control movement. Fortunately, neuropathy affecting motor control and muscle function is not too common. Symptoms of this kind are a reduction in muscle function, such as weakness in the arms and legs. Sometimes this results in an abnormal way of walking and misalignment of joints, mostly in the feet.

Neuropathy in the sensory system is another thing altogether. It is painful. It can also be a tingling, stabbing, burning sensation, or cause piercing pain, occurring mostly at night when you are trying to sleep.

The most common form of neuropathy in the sensory system is loss of feeling in the lower limbs. Insensitivity to touch occurs most often in the feet and legs, and much less often in the arms and hands. Although walking may not cause pain, the loss of feeling makes you unaware of any immediate damage to the foot. It is often after you remove your footwear that you discover that a foot ulcer has developed.

Neuropathy in the inner organs, namely, the autonomic nervous system, can give rise to dizziness, especially if you stand up too quickly. You may even experience nausea and vomiting after eating a meal. Other problems are diarrhoea, constipation, and difficulty in passing urine. A big problem for men is impotence, which can be very distressing – but not irreversible.

Prevention

Obviously, the best preventive measure against diabetic neuropathy is to keep the blood glucose levels as near normal as possible. Patients who are in a high-risk category should ask for treatment, such as regular foot care, professionally fitted shoes, and custom-made shoe inserts. It is important to remember that all persons with diabetes, even those without any risk factors, must be careful with their feet. You should make it a priority to ascertain your own individual risk status, and take action.

☐ Inspect your feet every day to avoid sores and ulcers. This is a very important as carelessness in this area could have very serious results.

☐ Make regular appointments to see a chiropodist for treatment of calluses, nails, hard skin, etc.

Diabetics who like to jog should be especially careful of their feet. There is a likelihood of infection should you get a blister while exercising. To bypass this possibility always wear comfortable running shoes. In fact wear them all the time. Try the mesh-vented shoes and specially designed athletic socks to soak up sweat and help prevent blisters in the first place.

Low intensity exercise before and after hard exercise

prevents injury. First it gradually increases your heart rate and blood pressure, then gently decreases them, making your workout easier on vulnerable blood vessels.

Treating Neuropathy With Medication

The most important aspect in treating neuropathy is controlling the blood glucose level and checking your feet daily to prevent the development of foot sores.

At present there is no medication to treat the reduced sense of touch.

Pain associated with touch can be controlled by medication such as:

- □ light painkillers (paracetamol or aspirin);
- □ light morphine-based drugs;
- □ in some cases with tricyclic anti-depressants.

Dizziness caused by standing up too quickly can quickly be overcome by wearing compression stockings.

Nausea and vomiting can be treated with various drugs known as anti-emetics.

Drugs can be taken for diarrhoea or in anticipation of events which might provoke an acute attack. Useful drugs include Diarrest, Lomotil, or Imodium.

Learning how to self-catheterise the bladder can be helpful for bladder problems.

Impotence can be treated with medication, such as 'Viagra'.

DIABETIC ACIDOSIS

Mellitus diabetes sufferers can usually avoid diabetic

acidosis by keeping to a strict regime of insulin treatment. This distressing condition can quickly occur if you fail to take your prescribed insulin doses. An infection is also known to be a factor in the onset of diabetic acidosis. Quite often it is triggered by another illness, and can develop over a period of time ranging from a matter of hours to few days.

As you are aware, the main function of insulin is to lower your blood glucose level, but, if your body lacks insulin, the blood glucose will rise. If the situation continues, and the insulin level drops significantly, then your body will go into an uncontrollable spiral and start burning fat instead of glucose. One thing leads to another and then glucose begins to show up in your urine, along with ketone bodies. Now the downward spiral really begins! Your body fluids begin to become too acidic due to the loss of glucose and ketone bodies. In a last ditch attempt to reduce the level of acid your rate and depth of breathing increases. At the same time, the high secretion of glucose into the urine causes the loss of large quantities of water and salts, putting your body at serious risk of dehydration. You will now find yourself suffering from a raging thirst, fatigue, increased urination and possibly confusion. If left too long it can lead to loss of consciousness.

Self Help

The most important thing is to prevent diabetic acidosis from developing in the first place. This is done by keeping tight control of your blood glucose levels. If you measure it regularly, you will notice any rises.

Early diagnosis is essential. If treated in the early stages you should recover fully within a few days. If you fail to get treatment, it will become life-threatening.

It is particularly important to measure your blood glucose level when you are not feeling well. If it is in double figures and you have any of the following problems seek medical advice quickly:

☐ Fast, deep breathing, even when you are not doing anything in particular.

☐ You have the smell of acetone on your breath.

☐ You keep feeling nauseous, begin vomiting and have stomach pains.

☐ If your blood glucose level is very high, you must measure the ketone bodies in your urine immediately. If you do detect ketone bodies, contact your doctor for help and advice.

☐ Remember to make sure that your ketone-measuring urine strips are recent as they go out of date very quickly. Using out of date strips do not always detect ketone bodies even if they are present.

☐ Avoid coming into contact with others who may be suffering from contagious infections. Diabetic acidosis is often preceded by an infection, such as a bronchial or stomach infection. Often an infection can lead to high levels of ketone bodies in the blood, known as 'ketoacidosis,' causing nausea, vomiting and loss of appetite. At its worst, it can cause lowered blood pH and possible heart failure and coma. Most sufferers make the mistake of believing that less insulin is needed when they are ill, but this is totally wrong. During a serious illness, especially during the presence of an infection with fever, more insulin is almost always necessary. In fact, taking less insulin when you need more because of the infection very quickly leads to diabetic ketoacidosis.

☐ To be on the safe side, always measure your blood glucose level if you are suffering from any kind of illness, and if the level is high, take more insulin to lower the glucose level.

☐ Don't embark on severe exercise to reduce high blood glucose levels and ketone bodies in the urine. Exercise will only makes matters worse. Remember, diabetic acidosis is caused by a low insulin level, and must be treated with insulin.

Orthodox Treatment

Once the diagnosis is made you will be treated in hospital on an in-patient basis, often in an Intensive Care Unit. Treatment consists of:

☐ Intravenous fluids, initially with salt-containing, and later glucose-containing fluids.

☐ Intravenous insulin infusion.

☐ Potassium supplements added to the infusion.

☐ Antibiotics, if an infection is identified.

☐ Carefully controlled exercise.

KETONE BODIES

Ketones are substances chemically related to acetone,

which is found in solvents such as nail polish remover. When your body is forced to burn body fat for energy, instead of glucose, fatty acids are released into the blood, where they are converted to ketones. Your body disposes of excess amounts of ketones by secreting them out of your body with your urine.

When you have a high blood glucose count (hyperglycaemia), or low blood glucose count (hypoglycaemia), ketones begin to appear in your blood. When you exercise, you use a lot of energy. If you have too little insulin and/or glucose during or after exercise, your body will burn fat, causing ketones.

Stress both mental and physical is a common element causing your body to need more glucose. If their isn't enough, your body will start burning fat for energy instead.

How Do I Know If I Have Ketones In My Urine?

If you have high blood glucose and/or have some symptoms from the list below you may have ketones. If you have high blood glucose levels, and your ketones are high for long periods of time, you could develop diabetic acidosis. Signs of diabetic acidosis or ketones in your urine, include:

☐ dry mouth;

☐ great thirst;

☐ fruity breath;

☐ loss of appetite;

☐ stomach pain;

☐ nausea;

☐ vomiting;

☐ dry, flushed skin;

☐ fever;

☐ fatigue;

☐ drowsiness;

☐ frequent urination;

☐ laboured breathing.

If you have these symptoms, or have a blood glucose level over 240 mg/dL, you should test your urine using a ketone test kit. Although there are several kinds, most people use the strips. These are just like your test strips but you get a sample of fresh urine on them, and wait for the product's specified time and match the colour on the chart on the bottle. It is a good idea to record all ketone tests along with your regular blood glucose counts, and insulin dosages. If you have large amounts of ketones in your urine, you should then contact your doctor immediately for further instruction. If you have a 'trace' or 'small' amount of ketones in your urine you should, drink a glass of water every hour and test your blood glucose every three hours. If blood glucose and ketone levels are not going down after two to three tests, call your doctor.

DIABETIC KIDNEY DISEASE

The kidneys are usually described as bean-shaped, being slightly narrower in the middle with bulging ends, much the same shape as a bean. These are ductless glands and are of great importance in the correct working of the body. Knowing the signs of kidney problems is important. The pain from kidney troubles is felt very typically in the back of the loins, and pressure there will sometimes relieve the pain temporarily. Perhaps the most common signs of trouble includes burning pain whilst urinating, frequent urination, blood in the urine, swelling of the hands and feet, pain in the back or side below the ribs, and high blood pressure.

Causes

Diabetic kidney disease is often associated with high blood pressure. So, if your blood pressure is constantly high, it's time for you to do something about it. Controlling blood pressure and protein levels in the urine is very important, as this can cause diabetic kidney disease in diabetics. High blood glucose levels are another major factor in this disease. It causes damage to the small blood vessels in the kidneys, released protein into the urine. It is also thought that diabetic kidney disease may also be associated with diabetic retinopathy.

If you think you may have problems don't worry, the disease can be detected through routine urine samples. Modern day treatment of diabetic kidney disease is much more advanced than in the past, when many patients needed dialysis or a kidney transplant.

Symptoms

Whilst the disease is developing you may be totally unaware that anything is wrong. Later however, the following signs of decreased kidney function can occur:

- ☐ Constant tiredness for no apparent reason.
- ☐ Feeling nauseous and/or vomiting.
- ☐ Uncontrolled itchy skin.

☐ A metallic taste in the mouth.
☐ Heartburn.
☐ Oedema in the limbs and/or eyelids.

Prevention

☐ The earlier you catch signs of kidney disease the better, so have your urine tested regularly for early signs of kidney disease. Your doctor may prescribe pills to delay more damage to your kidneys.

☐ High blood glucose levels increase the risk of developing diabetic kidney disease. For this reason it is essential to maintain a strict check on your blood glucose levels, and keep it as near normal as possible.

☐ Have your urine tested for signs of protein (albumin) at least once a year.

☐ Visit your doctor on a regular basis to have your blood pressure monitored.

☐ Drink up to 2 litres of liquid a day, especially when hot weather or activity increases perspiration.

☐ Empty your bladder as soon as you feel the need.

☐ Always consult your doctor about any kidney trouble, since it can become serious if ignored.

Chapter Five

Improving Your Health

ATHEROSCLEROSIS

The term means degeneration of the walls of the arteries due to the formation in them of fatty plaques and scar tissue. Nowadays, the name is now commonly applied to the general condition of a patient in whom this hardening of the arteries has occurred. The narrowing does not occur suddenly but builds up over several years where cholesterol fat and the smooth muscle cells lining the blood vessels have been transformed into a thickened and sometimes calcified mass. The result is that the arteries become constricted, their elasticity disappears and the volume of blood able to travel through them at any given time is reduced.

Atheroma affects a lot of people. It can start as early as the 20s and increases with age. The exact cause is unknown but several risk factors leading to atherosclerosis have been identified:

    □ a family history of atherosclerosis;

    □ smoking;

    □ diabetes type 1 & type 2;

    □ hypertension (high blood pressure);

    □ high content of cholesterol in the blood;

☐ being of the male gender;

☐ excess weight.

Prevention

There is no medication currently available to cure atherosclerosis. Nor are there any drugs available which can make constricted arteries regain their elasticity.

Some patients benefit from cholesterol lowering medicine which reduce the progression of disease and the likelihood of plaque rupture. Often medicine preventing thrombosis (blood clotting) is also given, such as acetylsalicylic acid (aspirin).

What can be done to prevent atherosclerosis?

If you suffer from diabetes type 1 or type 2 or high blood pressure ensure that treatment for these is maintained.

☐ Stop smoking. Your doctor or pharmacist will be able to provide advice and information on smoking cessation products and techniques.

☐ Eat a varied healthy diet, full of greens, fibre and, of course, low fat products. Avoid saturated fats found in red meat like pork and beef.

☐ Lose weight, if overweight.

☐ Exercise more. Half an hour walking a day is much better than nothing at all.

REDUCING CHOLESTEROL LEVELS

High cholesterol and other fats in the blood can lead to heart disease and stroke, so it is essential that you have your blood fats tested annually to check your triglyceride levels. If your cholesterol is high, you may need to change your diet and exercise habits, or take pills to keep your blood fats at healthy levels.

Triglyceride levels are an independent risk factor for coronary heart disease. This means that a person's risk for coronary heart disease is increased whenever triglyceride levels are high.

Abnormally high triglyceride levels may be due to:
□ chronic renal failure and other kidney diseases;
□ diabetes;
□ hypothyroidism, or an underactive thyroid gland;
□ inflammation of the pancreas, which in turn may be caused by high levels of triglycerides;
□ an inherited, impaired ability to process fats that results in high levels of fats in the blood;
□ medicines, including corticosteroids, oestrogen, and high doses of beta-blockers.

There are several things you can do to reduce your cholesterol levels, but it will take a good deal of will power. If you are overweight you must take notice of the diet prescribed for you. If you eat a lot of foods containing carbohydrates you may have to cut down if they are excessive. Smoking, drinking alcohol, and lack of exercise are all high on the list for increasing your cholesterol, so be forewarned and don't let it ruin your life.

Pecan Nuts And Cholesterol

According to a clinical study conducted by researchers

from California based Loma Linda University, eating pecan nuts may be a possible factor in helping to reduce blood cholesterol levels, provided they are consumed in conjunction with a healthy diet.

Their findings were published in the September issue of the *Journal of Nutrition*, in which they explained that by eating a traditional low fat diet with the addition of a daily amount of pecan nuts, the participants more than doubled their diet's cholesterol lowering effectiveness.

The clinical study was set-up under test conditions to see what would happen when volunteers consumed a low-fat diet prescribed for patients with high cholesterol levels, and a similar diet that replaced 20% of the calories with pecan nuts, added to dishes such as cereals and salads.

When publishing their findings, researchers said that the study group did not have any increase in body weight even though it actually contained 11% more fat.

Apple Juice

Researchers now tell us that there is some truth in the old saying "An apple a day keeps the doctor away!" Apparently, pure apple juice can do just that.

At the California-Davis University, researchers discovered that 'phyto-nutrients' (the active components in plants) in apple juice helps slow the oxidation of 'bad' (LDL) cholesterol that can lead to clogged arteries and heart disease.

Over a period of 12 weeks, 25 adults drank 1½ cupfuls of apple juice daily. That is equal to eating two apples per day. At the end of the period researchers found that the subjects consumption of apple juice slowed the detrimental LDL oxidation process. This first-ever clinical study of apple products, published in the *Journal of Medicinal Food,* is another reason why 100% apple juice and apple products should be among everyone's five daily servings of fruits and vegetables.

REDUCE YOUR RISK OF HIGH BLOOD PRESSURE

High blood pressure indicates that you are a candidate for eye disease, heart disease, stroke and kidney disease, so ask to have your blood pressure reading taken every 3 to 4 months. If it is high, you may need to speak to your dietician about changing your diet. You may also need to exercise more or take medication to reduce your blood pressure.

A healthy heart beats on average around 70 to 80 times a minute. It works in the same manner as a mechanical pump, driving oxygenated blood through the arteries out to various part of the body, which then returns to the heart to repeat the whole process over again. Another very important characteristic of the blood flowing through your body is pressure. Because the heart and your arteries are physically pushing the blood through and around your body, it is under a great deal of pressure. Blood pressure is expressed as millimetres of mercury (mm Hg). What this means is how high a column of mercury the pressure in your arteries could support. Two numbers are usually used that represent the pressure during systole and diastole respectively. A typical measurement might be written as 120/80. This is read as 'one-twenty over eighty'.

Just as blood flow varies at different locations, so does

blood pressure. In the aorta, nearest your heart, the pressure may be as high as 130 mm Hg. In your arm and also in a large artery but farther from your heart, it might be 110, and in the smaller vessels and capillaries it can be as low as 5 or 10. Venous blood pressure can even be less than zero.

Factors Affecting Blood Pressure

There are a number of risk factors linked to high blood pressure. Age is a major factor, many older people are more likely to develop high blood pressure, in particular if you are male. It is also more common in people with Afro-Caribbean origins. Other groups at risk include those with a family history of high blood pressure, heart disease or stroke. Other factors include being overweight, too much salt, a sedentary lifestyle, drinking too much alcohol, smoking and oral contraceptives may also contribute to raised blood pressure.

Many normal activities can cause variations in your blood pressure. These variations do not mean there is a problem. Your emotions, your physical position – whether you are sitting, lying, or standing, and even the time of day can affect your blood pressure. The table below list things that can either raise or lower your blood pressure.

CAUSE	CHANGE
Rest/Sleep	Lower
Evening	Higher
Morning	Lower
Anger	Higher
Excitement	Higher
Fear	Lower

CAUSE	CHANGE
Hot weather	Lower
After bath	Lower
Heavy meal	Higher
Exercise	Higher
Cold weather	Higher

Normal blood pressure for adults varies, but there is probably no problem if it is less than 140/90. High blood pressure indicates that the heart is working too hard. High blood pressure is bad for the heart and for arteries. Measurements above 140/90 mean a person has high blood pressure (hypertension) and should see a doctor. Hypertension can be an indication that a cycle of compensation and damage has begun that can lead to hardening of the arteries, kidney failure, heart attack, or stroke. In most cases, the doctor may not be able to identify a specific cause for the high blood pressure and will refer to it as essential hypertension. Fortunately, although the cause is not known, essential hypertension can be treated.

If you are diagnosed with high blood pressure, don't panic. If it is mild or moderate high blood pressure, you should make some changes in your lifestyle. If this doesn't help, your doctor may prescribe anti-hypersensitive medication.

If your doctor gives you medication to lower your blood pressure, it is important to take it regularly. If you find that it makes you feel unwell let your doctor know as there are several alternative treatments available.

Prevention

- ☐ Take part in regular activity. At least 30 minutes of brisk walking three to five times a week can make all the difference.
- ☐ Eat a healthy diet low in saturated fat and high in fibre, include five servings of fruit and vegetables per day.
- ☐ Reduce your salt intake. Avoid adding salt when cooking or at the table.
- ☐ Stop smoking.
- ☐ Lose any excess weight.
- ☐ Stick to recommended alcohol limits.

REDUCE YOUR RISK OF A STROKE

Stroke can affect anyone of any age, and it is people who have diabetes who run more than double the risk of stroke. That is because diabetics tend to suffer high blood pressure and furred up arteries, both of which increase the likelihood of stroke.

What Is A Stroke

A stroke happens when the blood supply to the brain is interrupted. Most strokes occur when a blood clot blocks an artery which is carrying blood to the brain. Some strokes are caused by bleeding within or around the brain from a burst blood vessel. When the blood supply is disrupted, the brain cells are deprived of oxygen and other nutrients, causing some cells to become damaged and other to die.

The Effects Of Stroke

Some strokes are fatal while others cause permanent or temporary disability. The most common effects of stroke are paralysis on one side of the body and loss of the ability to speak, read, or write.

Stroke Prevention

You can minimise your chance of stroke by making sure you pay attention to the risk factors which you can do something about. Factors which increase the risk of stroke fall into the following groups:

Lack of exercise – Start walking. This is the easiest, fastest, and perhaps cheapest form of exercise. Start slowly and begin with a 15 minute walk three times a week. Build up on this as you get stronger and increase your walks to 30 minutes. You want to condition yourself gradually, at the same time be careful not to get blisters and aching feet.

Drinking and Smoking – If you can't kick the habit, then at least cut down. A fast way to reduce your drinking is to order a single drink instead of a double, and then make it last. Smokers often have to try a variety of ways to quit before they find the one that works for them. fortunately, there are plenty of aids on the market that will help you stop smoking. A good method to stop is to keep both hands busy, that way you won't be able to hold a cigarette.

Overeating – Being too fat is linked to a number of health disorders, and stroke is high on the list. Work to reducing your consumption by starting the day as you mean to continue. When you are hungry it is much better to eat a piece of fruit or a drink of fruit or vegetable juice. When sitting down to eat a meal, drink a glass of water before you start, this will reduce your appetite.

RAPID RELIEF FOR CUTS AND SCRAPES

A cut or scrape can often be swollen and painful, but if it isn't serious enough to see your doctor then there is plenty you can do to help alleviate the pain and help it to heal quickly. The faster you can treat an injury, the better the chances are that it will heal properly, so make sure that you always have a first-aid kit available, whether in the home, at work, or in the car.

Keeping a wound moist with an airtight dressing can help it to heal faster than using gauze or other bandages. Doctors are not entirely sure why this should be, but it works very well. There are several types of airtight dressings made of polyurethane film. Each dressing is slightly different, but all have polyurethane exteriors with an interior layer of bio-compatible material that 'dissolves' into the wound. It should be noted, however, that airtight dressings are not suitable for chronic wounds such as diabetic sores.

Echinacea has potent immune-stimulating properties that help the body heal wounds. It can be taken as a drink to strengthen the immune system, or applied externally to the site of the wound.

Diabetes can cause the nerves that control sweating in your feet to no longer work. When this happens the skin of your feet becomes dry and scaly, and if not attended to your the skin may peel and crack.

To prevent injury, bathe your feet every day, and after bathing, dry your feet, and seal in the moisture that remains with a thin covering of plain petroleum jelly, unscented hand cream, or other such products. Do not put oils or creams between your toes. The extra moisture can lead to infection.

Foot calluses can be a big problem for diabetics, they very quickly become very thick, break down, and turn into ulcers. To keep them in check, use a wet pumice stone every day, and then massage your feet with a good foot lotion right after you use the pumice stone.

Ulcers usually appear on the ball of the foot, or on the bottom of the big toe. Ulcers on the sides of the foot are usually due to poorly fitting shoes. Remember, even if an ulcer doesn't hurt, it should be seen by your doctor right away, as neglect can result in an infection.

Myth

I have been told that I should only eat special diabetic foods!

Don't listen to idle gossip! You can get expert advice from your dietician, who will probably tell you that your dietary needs are the same as any other healthy person. The consumption of special, commercially produced diabetic foods is discouraged by the British Diabetic Association, who feel that the very existence of such products promotes the idea that diabetics cannot eat normally.

Chapter Six

Diabetes, Exercise and Weight Loss

It is well documented that obesity is often a cause of type 2 diabetes, and that exercise is important in controlling the development of both obesity and diabetes. However, over the last few decades the incidence of type 2 diabetes has increased rapidly in the western world, thus making the disease a major threat to public health.

A report in the *Archives of Internal Medicine* reveals that excessive television viewing is a significant indication of a sedentary lifestyle, thus making inactive people susceptible to both obesity and diabetes.

In 1986 Frank B. Hu, M.D. and a team of researchers from the Harvard School of Public Health, Harvard Medical School, and Brigham and Women's Hospital began a study investigating the lifestyles of nearly 38,000 men who were between 40 and 75 years old. To begin with, all of the subjects had to be healthy, and not suffering from diabetes, heart disease or cancer. Each subject was required to complete a questionnaire about their physical activity, smoking status, alcohol use, diet, television-viewing habits, and medical history. For the next 10 years, at two-year intervals, each subject completed a follow-up questionnaire which was then added to their dossier.

On completion of the study, the research team were in agreement that the more physically active men were less likely to smoke or be overweight or obese. It was also found that the most active men reduced their risk of developing diabetes by 53% compared to the least active.

When analysing the average number of hours spent watching TV each week, it became abundantly clear that persons who spent the most time watching TV were at a greater risk of developing diabetes. The report showed that viewers who watched TV for 21 to 40 hours per week were 77% more likely to get diabetes than those who watched for one hour per week. Worse still, those who viewed TV for over 40 hours per week were 120% more likely to get diabetes. These relationships took into account the men's body weight and various dietary characteristics such as consumption of cereal, fat, and red meat.

EXERCISE IS THE ONLY WAY

If the thought of exercising your body makes you feel depressed, then I sympathise with you. But, it's your body and your lifestyle that is deteriorating, and it's up to you to make that extra effort to do something about it! In adults, lack of adequate exercise is shown by comparative shortness of breath when carrying out physical tasks, the digestive tract becomes sluggish, the muscles become flabby, including the muscles of the heart, and you will probably suffer from bouts of constipation. It stands to reason, that in time health must suffer, and then the desire for taking exercise will be less. Thus a sort of vicious circle is established which can only be broken by a determined and systematic routine of exercise. Meanwhile, these unhealthy physical conditions affect the mental faculties. Worry, depression, and imaginary fears begin to obtrude, judgement becomes less sure, and decisions more difficult take.

All this is recognised by the medical profession, but when you think about it, the effect of exercise is obvious. There is an increased flow of blood to the working muscles, filling both the arteries and veins with blood within the muscles during exercise. This in turn nourishes the muscles and assists the body's metabolism. When you bring yourself to continue exercising regularly, your muscles will develop and the mobility of your joints will increase. One of the great merits of regular exercise is the comparative freedom from minor ailments which it confers. In addition it increases the stamina and the power of resistance to serious disease. It help banish worry, and imparts a sense of well being and enjoyment of life, so that the problems of life are tackled in that spirit of cheerful optimism which is more than half the battle, and helps a lot towards success.

There are of course other benefits attributable to exercise. If you are overweight, you will stand every chance of losing some of the excess baggage that you are carrying around. Believe me, it is only necessary to begin exercising more often and more intensely to reach a state of fitness that will make you feel stronger and more alert. If you are still interested, then the only other thing you have to do is find a form of exercise that you can enjoy, and then keep it up regularly.

Whether or not you need to lose weight, weight loss generally comes about when you exercise regularly and accompany it with a nourishing diet. In fact, diet is very important, because when you exercise, you burn calories, this alone makes it essential that you eat well-balanced meals to control your calorie consumption.

For those that have not been physically active for a long time, gentle, steady progress is the way forward. A good way to start is to carry on with your usual routine, but do thing in a way that requires a bit more energy. Then build these activities into your daily lifestyle.

If you were planning on losing weight but hadn't thought of including exercise, then think again. To achieve permanent weight loss, exercise is essential. A diet that is low in calories is risky for anyone, especially for those with diabetes.

The chances are, you are saying to yourself that exercise makes you feel hungry. But this is not the case. Often, the hungry feeling is just appetite stimulated by habit, which can be overcome in time if you continue to exercise. Exercise is the only way, combined with a good diet plan, to maintain weight loss and create a healthy body, and at the same time, reduce the amount of food that you eat. With a little help from your dietician, you should be able to adjust your diet plan so that you can exercise accordingly.

DIABETES, EXERCISE AND HYPOGLYCAEMIA

Diabetic sufferers should never underestimate the value of exercise. When exercising, glucose in the blood is put to use to provide energy, thereby lowering blood glucose levels. It also helps to delay or even stop heart (cardiovascular) disease. Unfortunately, cardiovascular disease is a leading killer of people with diabetes, making it all the more important for people with diabetes to exercise and counteract their increased risk of getting this deadly disease.

Control of your glucose levels whilst exercising is important, because the onset of hypoglycaemia is a very real risk. Because there is a risk, any regular exertion will mean that your diabetes care plan will need to be modified. This modification will reflect the correct balance of food, and insulin required for your additional physical activity. You and your dietician should work together to find out what is best for you.

AVOIDING INJURY

As with any exercise, and it doesn't matter whether it's organised exercise or just exercising at home, you must be careful that you don't hurt yourself. Don't ever forget, being diabetic makes you more vulnerable than others when something like a mediocre scratch becomes infected, or a pulled hamstring lays you up for a while. You can do two things to prevent injury to your muscles and sinews. First of all, gently stretch your muscles for a few minutes before you exercise. This will get your blood circulation moving and warm-up your muscles, making them supple for the main exercise you propose to do. Increase the length and intensity of exercise or activity gradually. When you finish exercising, repeat the gentle exercise for a few minutes to prevent your muscles cooling too rapidly and becoming stiff and achy. If you feel pain or uncomfortable stiffness after an activity, then you've overdone it. Secondly, you will need to gradually build up the intensity and duration of your exercise over many weeks or months. Don't try to do too much at once. You have to build up your strength and stamina slowly. Trying to do too much too soon will only tire you, making you wonder if it's all worthwhile

EFFECTS OF EXERCISE

Once you get into a regular workout routine, you will want to know if the exercise is doing you any good. I guess the first indication that the exercises are working is a reduction in the 'pot-belly' that most men are prone to get. Ladies may hope to see slimmer hips, thighs and tummy. Whatever your gender, you will without doubt see an improvement, but unfortunately the weighing scales may not confirm what you see. Whatever the exercise, whether it's jogging, walking, or exercising at a gymnasium, you will see the same benefit; a reduction in the amount of fat on your body and an increase in the strength of your muscles. And because your muscles have improved, you will feel the benefit.

Once you have built up your strength and stamina, it's worthwhile finding out how intense your workouts are, and to do this you need to count your pulse rate. To count your pulse rate, place your first two fingers (not your thumb) over the radial artery, which is found in the top third of your other wrist on the thumb side. Use light but firm pressure so that you can feel your pulse. Count the number of beats in 10 seconds immediately after you stop exercising. Don't delay, otherwise your heart slows down too quickly to get an accurate number. Multiply that number by 6 to get the number of heartbeats per minute.

If you feel that taking your pulse is a hit and miss affair, it might be provident to buy yourself a personal trainer LCD watch. It's the ideal aid to getting fit and keeping fit. These watches are capable of being used as a pedometer, as well as giving a readout of the average calories consumed. Another gadget is the heart rate monitor. They will measure and display your heart rate whilst exercising using a digital readout, thus providing you with a safe and effective method of continuously checking your heart rate whilst exercising.

Getting Started

Before you start participating in sports or other energetic exercises it would be a sensible precaution to ask your doctor to give you a thorough medical examination. This is the only way to make sure you are physically up to participating in the exercise that you have chosen.

No rules can be laid down for the amount of exercise taken as everyone is different, and your exercise plan needs to be based on your health and your body's needs. Your staying power, and state of health is the safest guide. You should feel that you have done enough, but still have the confidence of knowing that you're doing all you can to avoid any pitfalls and reap only the benefits of exercise.

Time For Exercise

Exercise shouldn't be taken just after a meal because the exercise will draw blood to the muscles being worked. This action will deplete other parts of the body, including the stomach which needs a full supply of blood during the earlier stages of digestion. Also, owing to the position of the stomach in the body, once it is distended by a full meal, it may press on the heart during physical exercise.

Another point that is not so well known, is that strenuous exertion just before or after a meal lowers the normal acidity of the stomach's gastric secretions, and affects the muscular action of the stomach wall, thus impairing digestion. On the other hand, light exercise after an ordinary meal may tone up the stomach, and stimulate its secretions. In summing up, it seems that a leisurely walk after a meal is good for you, but it is best to wait for at least three-quarters of an hour after finishing a meal before starting strenuous exercising.

TYPES OF EXERCISE

There is no restriction in the kind of exercise or sport a diabetics can participate in, though I would draw the line at boxing or similar type of combative contesting. The best way to test your stamina is to set some realistic goals for yourself. For example, you might find that a simple walk around the block for 15 minutes a day is enough. After a week or so you may want to build up on the time you are out walking, and set new goals in order to stay motivated. Walking is a most useful exercise because it costs nothing, calls into play many important muscles, and can be graduated to suit your individual pace, route and distance. A gentle stroll on the level may afford ample exercise for a person who is not strong, while another can indulge in a long cross-country ramble.

If you don't like walking on your own, get someone to go with you. When we exercise by ourselves we sometimes feel isolated and lose interest. However, a companion often provides the necessary encouragement and motivation to help us succeed. It also helps if you both have similar goals so that you can exercise at the same level. A training partner who is aware of your diabetes can also keep your exercise sessions safer for you.

Dancing is an excellent form of mild exercise with the advantage that rhythm and balance are cultivated. Swimming is also an extremely good exercise for those with whom bathing is pleasurable, it develops a healthy circulation, and induces deep breathing, and helps to develop the chest and heart muscles.

Stair-climbers and treadmills are excellent machines to use at the gym. They simulate walking and climbing which can help burn fat, build endurance, and strengthen the cardiovascular system. Weight-lifting can also provide a great workout. The important thing is to find something you enjoy, and exercise safely. Riding a stationary bicycle not only gives you a great aerobic workout, but it also strengthens your legs and helps build muscular endurance.

Age Impediments

Age should be no barrier to exercise. For the middle-aged golf is an ideal form of exercise. It takes place out of doors, it involves many co-ordinated movements, and it can be carried out as vigorously or as leisurely as desired. If it is difficult to get out and about there is still much you can do in your own home, such as stretching exercises. These can be done, either while standing or sitting. As our bodies age, warming up with stretching exercises becomes more and more important. You may find that after moderate stretching, you can do more than you thought you could.

EXERCISE AND DEHYDRATION

It is especially important for diabetics to prevent dehydration and to replenish the fluids and nutrients the body loses during exercise. As a precaution always make sure that you have a plentiful supply of water available with you. Drink at least one glass of water before you begin your exercise, and another glassful when you finish. If needed, take a drink as often as necessary whilst exercising as well. During strenuous exercise, consider a high-glucose sports drink which can help prevent your blood sugar from going too low.

Myth

My parents say that taking part in sports activities is dangerous, even though I say I'll be alright. How can I convince them that exercise is good for diabetics?

There are many ways. First, you should ask your parents to talk to your paediatrician and ask them what you can and cannot do. Secondly, you could talk with another parent of a child with diabetes and find out which sport(s) their child plays.

Make them aware of the many leading sports participants who are diabetic, and take part in their chosen sport year after year. Tell them about Sir Steve Redgrave, the winner of five Olympic gold medals for rowing. Then there is the professional athletes with diabetes such as NFL Quarterback Wade Wilson and 1950s tennis star Bill Talbert. That should convince them that exercise is OK.

Exercise as an essential part of maintaining a healthy lifestyle. It is a well known fact that keeping active will help you to avoid complications associated with diabetes, such as heart disease.

Of course care should be taken if you rely on insulin injections or have to take certain tablets. But being careful will help to avoid having a low blood glucose level when doing strenuous exercise. Always carry a high-sugar snack with you in case your blood glucose levels fall too low, and you may need to reduce your insulin dose. It is a good idea to discuss strenuous exercise with your doctor before embarking on any new exercise plan.

Chapter Seven

Travel Tips

Touring abroad or within the UK, particularly if it is a holiday, does the mind and body a power of good, relieving you of stresses that the daily grind brings to us all. But, to make any journey successful, whether on holiday or out of necessity, planning ahead is the key to arriving safely at your destination. And this is particularly true for people with diabetes – a little forethought will take you a long way and help keep you healthy once you are there. Whether you want to ramble over the Yorkshire Dales, visit the lakes of Cumbria, or lie on the beach in the Costa del Sol sunshine, you must ensure that you make allowances for the changes in your routine.

Plan To Avoid Stress

Just because you have diabetes it shouldn't stop you from doing the things you want to do, and touring is one of those things. If you want to see the world, and you have diabetes, just a little planning before you start your journey will make all the difference. Of course travelling can be physically and mentally tiring at times, especially when things go wrong. Most of us have experienced a delayed departure, or had our baggage lost at some foreign location, and no matter who it is, it always sends the blood pressure soaring, and raising the blood glucose levels. But, when it happens to you, there are things you must do, so be prepared before you leave your home or hotel room, and avoid any undue stress.

CHOOSING A TRAVEL OPERATOR

When making travel arrangements, whether it is by land, sea, or air, explain to the operator's representative that you have diabetes, and make sure they understand your particular needs whilst on their transport. In this way, an appropriate itinerary can be planned to meet your needs. On no account use an operator that fails to give you an assurance that your needs can be catered for. In this day and age, there are so many operators in the travel industry that you can afford to pick and choose.

VACCINATIONS AND MEDICATIONS

Make arrangements to get any required vaccinations at least six weeks before you travel, this will give you time to get over any possible side effects. Next port of call is your doctor's surgery where you should make arrangements to see your doctor for a check-up; this should be done at least four weeks before you travel. If you have a health care nurse, work out with him/her, any changes you may need for your meals and medication. This is especially important if you are travelling through different time zones.

Ask your doctor or health care nurse for a list of your medications. The list should include the generic names of your medication, and the dosage specifically applicable to you. If you take insulin, record the types of insulin and whether the insulin is short, intermediate or long-acting. Make a copy of the list, a photocopy will do, and carry one copy with you at all times.

Carrying medicines, syringes and needles in some countries can present a problem when entering the country. Depending on where you are travelling to, it may be expedient to obtain a written document from your doctor, stating that you are allowed to carry medicines or supplies.

Carry Identification

If the worst scenario happens and you become incoherent or unconscious, you will need some identification with you that explains your condition. You may already have it, but if not, consider getting a MedicAlert™ bracelet or necklace that states that you have diabetes. You should also carry a card detailing your type of diabetes and the treatment you require. Medic Alert is the Emergency Identification System for people with hidden medical conditions which place them at risk. You can obtain a membership form by writing to:

Medic Alert, 1 Bridge Wharf, 156 Caledonian Road, London N1 9UU, or phone 020 7833 3034

TRAVEL INSURANCE

Some insurance plans do not cover pre-existing medical conditions, which includes diabetes, consequently it has been a struggle in the past to find adequate insurance cover. Even when cover has been provided it is prohibitively expensive, and applicants are made to have more than one medical.

That is now all set to change, because the charity Diabetes UK has organised a new partnership with the leading health insurance broker Heath Lambert, to provided insurance policies for people with diabetes. The policies will cover travel, motor and home insurance cover, and cover complications that could arise from diabetes.

Heath Lambert staff are trained by Diabetes UK, and can be contacted on a freephone number, 0800 731 7431.

PACKING

Think ahead when packing your medications. Take extra supplies and medication in case of loss, theft or accidental destruction. With the increasing numbers of people travelling nowadays there is always someone who loses their baggage, albeit it is left behind, or sent to the wrong destination. In the event that it's your luggage that is lost, it could be a disaster in the making if you can't get fresh supplies right away. So, be smart and pack your medications and diabetes supplies in separate bags, making sure that some of them are in your hand-luggage. In this way, you will at least have some of your supplies with you. Don't forget to include other medications you may need, such as treatment for hypoglycaemia, nausea and diarrhoea. Also, make sure that you have adequate food supplies, drinking water, walking shoes, and sun-cream.

Myth

I want to learn to drive, but I am told I must not drive because I have diabetes.

If you are a responsible person and keep good control of your diabetes then you present no more danger on the roads than anyone else. However, it is difficult to convince people in authority that diabetics are safe on the road. To overcome this misconception, the charity Diabetes UK that funds research, is currently running a campaign to change legislation that prevents diabetics who treat their diabetes with insulin from driving certain vehicles.

THE TRAVELLER'S CHECKLIST

Before you leave:

- ☐ Have any needed vaccinations six weeks in advance.
- ☐ Have a medical check-up four weeks in advance.
- ☐ Arrange your travel health insurance.
- ☐ Obtain an identification card and MedicAlert™ bracelet or necklace.
- ☐ Compose a list of your medications.
- ☐ Obtain a letter from your doctor.
- ☐ Obtain information on local medical facilities or organisations where you are going to be.
- ☐ Make a note of your doctor's telephone number.

Ask your doctor or hospital diabetologist about:

- ☐ hypoglycaemia management (glucagon for insulin users);
- ☐ avoiding illness caused by contaminated food and water;
- ☐ tips for adjusting your medication if required.

Packing List:

- ☐ Pack extra food to cover delayed meals such as a box of biscuits or crackers and fruit juice.
- ☐ Pack fast-acting sugar to treat low blood glucose.
- ☐ Pack an extra supply of insulin or oral agent for diabetes.
- ☐ Pack an extra supply of syringes, needles and an extra insulin pen if used.
- ☐ Pack fast-acting insulin for high blood glucose and ketones.
- ☐ Pack a blood glucose testing kit and record book.
- ☐ Pack urine ketone-testing strips.
- ☐ Pack anti-nausea and anti-diarrhoea pills.
- ☐ Pack pain relieving medication.
- ☐ Pack sun-screen cream.
- ☐ Pack insect repellent.
- ☐ Pack large amounts of bottled water, if going to a hot country.
- ☐ Pack comfortable walking shoes, if you intend to go touring on foot.
- ☐ Pack glucagon.
- ☐ Pack supplies for the trip home, in case you run into any problems.

Myth

I thought it was only elderly people who were given flu jabs each year, so why have I been advised to attend the flu jab clinic?
The fact is, diabetics are no more likely to get flu or any

another illness. However, diabetic sufferers are advised to get flu jabs because any infection interferes with your blood glucose control, thus putting you at risk of high blood glucose levels. Also, sufferers of type 1 diabetes, have an increased risk of ketoacidosis if they catch an infection.

"Clean your arteries – it could save your life"

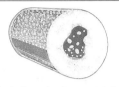

1. A clogged artery restricting the flow of blood

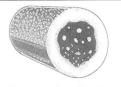

2. The artery is gradually cleaned, improving circulation

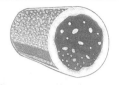

3. A clean artery allows full, healthy circulation

By Johnathon E. Briggs E.L.S.

Heart disease is the UK's number one killer – and one of the main causes is clogged arteries. Johnathon Briggs the author of a new book Clean your arteries – it could save your life has identified how clogged arteries can cause:

• Chest pain • dizziness • shortness of breath • high blood pressure • tired and painful legs • high cholesterol • poor circulation • poor balance and ringing in the ears • if you have any of those symptoms you could be at risk – but luckily for all of us Mr. Briggs now believes it is possible to reverse the damage already done using a very simple method and by following his method, not only will it clean your arteries, it could even save your life.

His new method along with hundreds of other tips and secrets that can help clean arteries are found in his remarkable new book *Clean your Arteries – it could save your life.*

It is widely recognised that people who have a healthy lifestyle have more energy, feel great every day, eat well, sleep soundly and even have better powers of concentration. *Clean your arteries – it could save your life* shows you a method that will change your lifestyle to a healthy one. Best of all, if you use this method, there is no need to invest in expensive equipment or make any major lifestyle changes. There is no rigorous exercise and not even an exotic diet. In fact it is surprisingly simple how easy it is to modify existing habits.

Here are just a few examples of the tips and secrets Mr. Briggs reveals in his remarkable new book

• The "power vitamins" that may protect you against heart disease
• The hidden dangers of some popular "healthfoods"
• The "organic" foods that could help you lose weight
• The "myth" of a low-fat diet
• A simple trick to prevent stress and anxiety

Plus much, much more.

The health of your arteries is very important – Don't waste time, send today for your copy of *Clean your arteries – it could save your life*. You have a full three months to try the book. If you are not completely satisfied, simply return it for a full refund. Get all the facts.

To Order

Call our freephone orderline on **0870 225 5010** or send your payment of £9.95 plus £1.95 p&p (payable to Windsor Health) or credit/debit card details including your card number, start date, expiry date and issue number for Switch together with your name, address and book title to:

**Windsor Health,
Dept DB1,
Emery House,
Brunel Road, Totton,
Southampton
SO40 3SH**

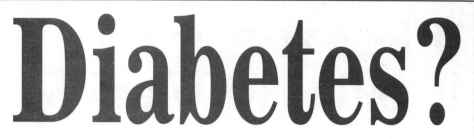

Diabetes?

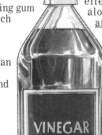